Simplified Solution Approach

To

HYPERTHYROIDISM

Unlocking Vitality: A Comprehensive Guide
to Restoring Hormonal Harmony and
Reclaiming Your Energy

Dr QUENTIN GLYN

Table Of Contents

CHAPTER ONE

Hyperthyroidism

A medical disease known as hyperthyroidism is characterized by an overactive thyroid gland that produces an excessive amount of thyroid hormones. These hormones are essential for controlling the body's metabolism, and high amounts of them may cause a number of symptoms and medical issues. Controlling hyperthyroidism is crucial to preventing further health problems and improving the general health of those who are impacted by this illness.

A Synopsis Of Hyperthyroidism

Thyroxine (T4) and triiodothyronine (T3) are two hormones that are produced by the thyroid gland, which is situated in the neck. These hormones are essential for controlling the body's metabolism. The hyperactive thyroid gland causes an excessive release of these hormones into the circulation in hyperthyroidism. A variety of symptoms, such as worry, weariness, heat intolerance, weight loss, and elevated heart rate, might be brought on by this enhanced hormonal activity.

An autoimmune condition called Graves' disease is often the cause of hyperthyroidism. Thyroid nodules, thyroiditis, or inflammation of the thyroid gland, and several drugs are other possible reasons. Untreated hyperthyroidism may lead to major side effects including osteoporosis, cardiac issues, and, in extreme situations, a potentially fatal disease called thyroid storm.

The Value Of An Approach To Simplified Solutions:

The management of hyperthyroidism necessitates a thorough and intelligible approach to solutions. The medical jargon, available treatments, and lifestyle changes may be too much for many people with this ailment. In order to enable patients to take an active role in their healthcare journey and successfully comply with recommended treatments, a simple solution approach is essential.

Simplifying the process not only helps people comprehend the nature of hyperthyroidism but also improves communication between patients and healthcare professionals. People may make educated choices regarding their treatment plans, lifestyle changes, and general well-being when complicated medical ideas are reduced to understandable and accessible information.

Objective And Range Of The Book:

The book aims to provide people with hyperthyroidism and those who support them with a clear, concise manual for understanding, treating, and leading fulfilling lives with this illness. The book seeks to provide people with practical activities they may take to enhance their quality of life, explain medical jargon, and clarify treatment alternatives.

The Book's Purview Includes:

Understanding Hyperthyroidism: Providing information on the causes, signs, and diagnosis of hyperthyroidism in a manner that is understandable to those with different backgrounds in medicine.

Treatment alternatives: Outline the possible advantages and disadvantages of each treatment choice, as well as discuss the variety of alternatives that are available, such as drugs, radioactive iodine therapy, and surgery.

Lifestyle Modifications: Offering helpful guidance on food restrictions, stress reduction techniques, and exercise regimens that may supplement medical therapies.

Managing Healthcare: Providing direction on how to communicate with medical professionals in an efficient manner, comprehend test findings, and speak out for one's own medical needs.

Emotional Well-Being: Handling the emotional effects of hyperthyroidism and offering coping mechanisms to handle sadness, anxiety, and other mental health issues related to the disease.

This book seeks to enable people with hyperthyroidism to actively participate in their health management via the adoption of a simple solution approach, which should improve results and enhance quality of life.

CHAPTER TWO

Comprehending Hyperthyroidism

Meaning And Reasons:

Thyroxine (T4) and triiodothyronine (T3) are the two main thyroid hormones that are overproduced by the thyroid gland in hyperthyroidism. These hormones are essential for controlling how the body uses energy. Excessive amounts of these may cause a number of symptoms as well as other health issues.

Reasons:

Graves' Disease: The most prevalent cause of hyperthyroidism is this autoimmune illness. When the thyroid gland is wrongly attacked by the immune system, it is stimulated to create additional hormones.

Toxic Nodular Goiter: When the thyroid gland develops nodules, the body produces too much hormone because the nodules don't follow the body's rules.

Subacute Thyroiditis: Thyroid inflammation, often brought on by a viral infection, results in a brief elevation in thyroid hormone levels.

Excessive Iodine: Hyperthyroidism may result from consuming an excessive amount of iodine via food or medicine.

Thyroiditis: When the thyroid becomes inflamed, the gland may release hormones that have been held in the circulation, temporarily raising the body's thyroid function.

Signs And Prognosis:

Signs:

Increased Metabolism: difficulties gaining weight, hyperactivity, and weight loss despite increased hunger.

Palpitations, elevated heart rate, and elevated blood pressure are symptoms of cardiovascular disease.

Effects of the Nervous System: Tremors, anxiety, impatience, and trouble focusing.

Muscle and Joint Problems: Weariness, weakness, and atrophy of the muscles.

Heat intolerance: The inability to tolerate warm weather.

Menstrual Changes: Women who have irregular menstrual periods.

Conclusion:

Blood Tests: Thyroid hormone (T3, T4) and thyroid-stimulating hormone (TSH) levels may be measured to aid in the diagnosis of hyperthyroidism.

Test for Radioactive Iodine Uptake: This test gauges the thyroid's activity by measuring the amount of radioactive iodine it absorbs.

Thyroid Scan: A radioactive isotope scan is used to determine the thyroid gland's size and functionality.

Physical Examination: Physicians may look for physical indicators of Graves' disease, such as abnormalities in the eyes (exophthalmos), and indicators of an enlarged thyroid (goiter).

Effect On General Health:

1. Heart System:

Elevated Heart Rate: Heart strain caused by hyperthyroidism may result in palpitations and a higher chance of arrhythmias.

High Blood Pressure: One of the most prevalent symptoms is elevated blood pressure.

2. Weight and Metabolism:

Weight Loss: People may find it difficult to maintain or gain weight while having a higher hunger because of a faster metabolism.

Muscular Wasting: The disintegration of muscular tissue may result from the elevated metabolic rate.

3. Mental Wellness:

Anxiety and Irritability: When thyroid hormone levels are too high, the neural system is impacted, which may cause elevated feelings of anxiety and emotion.

Difficulty Concentrating: Cognitive processes that affect memory and concentration may be compromised.

4. The reproductive system

Menstrual irregularities: Women may have problems conceiving as well as irregular periods.

5. Bone Well-being:

Osteoporosis Risk: Prolonged hyperthyroidism raises the possibility of fractures by causing a decrease in bone density.

6. Additional Difficulties:

Thyroid Storm: intense instances of uncontrolled hyperthyroidism may result in a thyroid storm, a potentially fatal illness marked by an abrupt and intense onset of symptoms.

To sum up, comprehending hyperthyroidism entails being aware of its origins, figuring out how to diagnose its symptoms, and realizing how it affects many facets of general health. For those with hyperthyroidism to avoid problems and have a higher quality of life, early diagnosis and treatment are essential.

CHAPTER THREE
Conventional Therapy Methods

Drugs Used To Treat Hyperthyroidism:

Antithyroid pharmaceuticals: Methimazole and propylthiouracil (PTU) are two of the antithyroid pharmaceuticals that are most often used for hyperthyroidism. These medications function by preventing the thyroid gland from producing thyroid hormones.

Beta-Blockers: Although they don't directly treat thyroid hormone levels, beta-blockers, such as propranolol, are often used to treat symptoms including anxiety, tremors, and a fast heartbeat.

Advantages:

Non-intrusive.

May provide symptomatic assistance.

Often the first course of action.

Cons:

Might not provide a long-term fix.

Consequences of antithyroid medications.

It is possible to relapse after stopping.

Therapy Using Radioactive Iodine:

When oral radioactive iodine is consumed, the thyroid gland absorbs it. Hormone synthesis is decreased because the radiation kills the hyperactive thyroid cells.

Advantages:

Non-intrusive.

High rate of effectiveness in lowering thyroid activity.

Usually a single treatment.

Cons:

may eventually result in hypothyroidism, or an underactive thyroid.

Unsuitable for ladies who are expecting.

Actions must be taken to prevent radiation exposure to other people.

Options For Surgery
(Thyroidectomy):

Another alternative is to surgically remove all or a portion of the thyroid gland, especially if previous therapies are not appropriate or successful.

Advantages:

offers a solution that is more rapid.

No continuous medication or radioactive iodine treatment is required.

may serve as a long-term fix.

Cons:

inherent dangers associated with surgery.

Possible harm to adjacent anatomical structures such as parathyroid glands.

Potential for hypothyroidism to develop after surgery.

Benefits and Drawbacks of Traditional Treatments

Drugs:

Advantages:

quick start of the action.

generally accepted favorably.

Cons:

Recurrence is frequent after cessation.

adverse effects include liver issues, joint discomfort, and dermatitis.

Therapy Using Radioactive Iodine:

Advantages:

high rate of achievement.

non-invasive method.

Cons:

Hypothyroidism risk.

Unsuitable for certain demographics.

Surgical Solutions:

Advantages:

Possibility of an enduring resolution.

lowering of thyroid hormone levels right away.

Cons:

hazards associated with surgery.

Hypothyroidism long-term danger.

It is important to remember that the selection of therapy is based on a number of variables, such as the degree of hyperthyroidism, the underlying reason, the age of the patient, and general health. Individual preferences, as well as the possible advantages and disadvantages of any therapy, should be carefully evaluated in conjunction with medical specialists. Over time, new treatment options may be introduced or current ones may be modified due to advancements in medical research.

CHAPTER FOUR

The Drawbacks Of Traditional Methods

Constraints Of Traditional Treatments For Hyperthyroidism:

Medications, radioactive iodine therapy, or, in extreme situations, surgery are the usual treatments for hyperthyroidism. These techniques do have significant drawbacks, even though they have helped a lot of people.

Inadequate Reduction of Symptoms: Reduction of symptoms may not always be achieved in full with traditional therapy.

Even after receiving conventional therapy, some patients may have lingering symptoms including tiredness, weight gain, or mood swings.

Relapse Rates: Although therapies for hyperthyroidism may not provide a long-term cure, relapses are possible. For example, a relapse of hyperthyroidism may occur in patients receiving medicine or radioactive iodine treatment, necessitating further measures.

Individual Variability in Response: There might be a wide range in a patient's reaction to traditional therapy. While some people may respond well to medicine, others may not get enough relief or even have negative side effects.

Consequences And Hazards:

Medication Side Effects: Methimazole and propylthiouracil, two anti-thyroid drugs, may have adverse effects that include rash, nausea, and in rare instances, more severe disorders including agranulocytosis. During the medication's titration, patients may also suffer variations in thyroid hormone levels, which might result in episodes of hypo- or hyperthyroidism.

Risks associated with radioactive iodine treatment include radiation exposure. Temporary neck pain or swelling is possible, and long-term hypothyroidism needing lifetime thyroid hormone replacement is a possibility.

Complications from Surgery: Thyroidectomy, or surgical removal of the thyroid gland, carries a risk of bleeding, infection, general anesthesia, and harm to surrounding tissues, including the parathyroid glands, which control calcium levels.

Difficulties With Long-Term Management:

Thyroid Hormone Fluctuations: It may be difficult to reach and maintain ideal thyroid hormone levels, especially while using medication. Hormone fluctuations may cause long-lasting symptoms and need regular dose changes for medications.

Monitoring and Follow-Up: Patients may find it difficult to undergo the frequent thyroid function monitoring required for the long-term therapy of hyperthyroidism. Successful management requires regular follow-up and adherence to treatment programs.

Problems with Quality of Life: Treatments for hyperthyroidism may have an adverse effect on quality of life. Issues with exhaustion, weight fluctuations, and emotional stability are common among patients and may not go away even after the hyperthyroidism is managed.

Views Of Patients Regarding Conventional Therapies:

Wish for Non-Invasive Treatments: A number of patients indicate that they would rather not have surgery or radioactive iodine therapy. This desire is often motivated by worries about long-term implications and possible adverse effects.

Effect on Daily Life: Conventional therapies have the potential to interfere with routine activities, especially when it comes to radioactive iodine therapy, which necessitates temporary seclusion. Patients may seek therapy with fewer restrictions on their lifestyle if they find these interruptions difficult.

Need for Personalized Approaches: Patients often want more individualized treatment regimens that take into account their particular symptoms, interests, and way of life. While many people find success with traditional therapies, they may not address the unique differences in how hyperthyroidism manifests and affects a person.

In conclusion, while traditional methods have been essential in treating hyperthyroidism, they are not without drawbacks, and patient input is vital in determining how future therapeutic techniques will be developed. Research developments and the creation of more specialized and customized methods have the potential to solve these issues and enhance the general treatment of hyperthyroidism.

CHAPTER FIVE
Changes In Lifestyle

Combining medication with lifestyle changes is common in the management of hyperthyroidism. This is a detailed summary of the lifestyle changes with an emphasis on how nutrition, exercise, stress reduction, and sleep are related to hyperthyroidism.

Adjustments To Lifestyle For Hyperthyroidism:

1. Dietary Adjustments:

a. Iodine Intake: - Steer clear of Excessive Iodine: Overindulging in iodine may worsen hyperthyroidism, which is often linked to an overactive thyroid. It is important to limit the intake of foods high in iodine, such as seaweed, iodized salt, and certain shellfish.

b. Essential Nutrients: Make sure your diet is well-balanced and contains important nutrients including zinc, omega-3 fatty acids, and selenium. These nutrients help to lower inflammation and maintain thyroid function.

c. Goitrogens may interfere with thyroid function, thus it's important to consume cruciferous vegetables in moderation. Broccoli and cabbage are examples of cruciferous vegetables that contain goitrogens. Even though these meals are nutritious, moderation is advised while consuming them.

2. Physical Activity And Stress Reduction:

a. Frequent Exercise: - Moderate Aerobic Activity: Take up cycling, swimming, or walking as examples of moderate aerobic workouts. Frequent exercise may improve general health and assist in controlling metabolism.

b. Strength Training: - Muscle Building: To increase lean muscle mass, include strength training activities. This may speed up metabolism and help with weight control, which is important for those with hyperthyroidism.

c. Stress Reduction Strategies: - Mindfulness and Relaxation: Prolonged stress may exacerbate the symptoms of hyperthyroidism. To encourage relaxation, engage in stress-reduction practices including mindfulness, meditation, and deep breathing exercises.

d. Yoga and Tai Chi: - Gentle Exercise Forms: These low-impact activities include both movement and awareness. They may help with stress reduction and balance promotion in general.

3. The Effects Of Sleep On Thyroid Health:

a. Regular Sleep Plan: - Make Quality Sleep a Priority: Create a regular sleep plan and strive for seven to nine hours of good sleep every night. Getting enough sleep is essential for good health in general and for controlling the synthesis of hormones, especially thyroid hormones.

b. Sleep hygiene: - Establish a Calm Environment: Reduce light and noise to create a pleasant sleeping environment. Minimize the amount of time spent on screens before bed since blue light exposure may disrupt the hormones that trigger sleep.

c. Handling Insomnia: - Relaxation Techniques: If you're having trouble sleeping, try progressive muscle relaxation or guided imagery as a way to unwind before bed.

Including these lifestyle changes in the hyperthyroidism management strategy may improve general health and enhance medication interventions. People with hyperthyroidism must collaborate closely with medical providers to customize these lifestyle modifications to their unique requirements and medical conditions. Whenever you make big dietary or activity changes, always get medical advice first, particularly if you have a thyroid condition.

CHAPTER SIX

Complementary And Integrative Therapies

A medical disease known as hyperthyroidism is characterized by an overactive thyroid gland that produces an excessive amount of thyroid hormones.

While antithyroid drugs and radioactive iodine therapy are the most often recommended conventional medical treatments for hyperthyroidism, some people also look into alternative and integrative therapies. It's important to remember that these methods shouldn't take the place of conventional medical care and should be explored with a healthcare provider. We'll explore integrative and complementary treatments in this section, with particular attention on acupuncture, herbal medicines and supplements, alternative therapies, and mind-body practices.

Supplements And Herbal Remedies:

1. (Lycopus europaeus) bugleweed:

Mechanism: Said to prevent the generation of thyroid hormones.

usage caution: Seek advice from a healthcare professional as prolonged usage may cause hypothyroidism.

2. Melissa officinalis (lemon balm):

Benefits: Known for its relaxing qualities, it might aid in reducing hyperthyroidism-related symptoms including anxiety.

Considerations: Interacts with certain drugs; thus, it is imperative to speak with a healthcare provider.

3. (Withania somnifera) ashwagandha:

Mechanism: This adaptogenic herb may have actions that modulate the thyroid.

Be cautious while checking thyroid levels, particularly in those who are hypothyroid.

4. Supplements with Iodine:

Role: Low iodine levels are common in hyperthyroidism patients, but supplementing has to be done with caution since high iodine levels might make the disease worse.

Acupuncture And Complementary Medicine:

1. Acupuncture

Benefits: Said to enhance general well-being and harmonize the body's energy, or Qi.

Exercise caution: Only have this done by a qualified and experienced acupuncturist.

2. Chiropractic Treatment:

Role: May aid in promoting overall well-being and addressing related musculoskeletal problems.

Be careful: Make sure the chiropractor is aware of the thyroid issue.

3. Homeopathic medicine:

Method: Tailored care according to the patient's unique symptoms.

Be cautious: For individualized treatment, speak with a qualified homeopath.

Mind-Body Methodologies:

1. Yoga:

Benefits include less stress, more flexibility, and maybe even better thyroid function.

Exercise caution: Although vigorous types of yoga are normally advised, they may have the opposite effect.

2. Practice meditation:

Role: Inducing relaxation and reducing stress.

Be cautious: Consistent practice is essential; expert instruction might be helpful.

3. Biofeedback:

Mechanism: Educates people on how to regulate their body's processes, maybe including the thyroid.

Be careful: Needs instruction from a certified professional.

Crucial Points To Remember:

Assisted by Healthcare Providers:

When using integrative treatments, always let healthcare practitioners know about them to guarantee a thorough and well-coordinated approach.

Frequent Observation:

Maintain routine testing for thyroid function to evaluate the effects of integrative therapies and modify treatment plans as needed.

Customized Method:

Understand that different people may respond to integrative treatments in different ways and that what works for one person may not work for another.

Prioritizing Safety

Make sure these treatments are safe, taking into account any pre-existing medical issues and any drug combinations.

To sum up, an integrative strategy for treating hyperthyroidism that includes acupuncture, herbal remedies, alternative therapies, and mind-body methods can offer a comprehensive approach to symptom management and enhance general health. To guarantee the security and efficacy of these complementary therapies when used in combination with traditional medical treatments, it is essential to collaborate closely with medical specialists.

CHAPTER SEVEN

Tailored Plans Of Care For Hyperthyroidism

A disease known as hyperthyroidism occurs when the thyroid gland generates an excessive quantity of thyroid hormones, which may cause anxiety, fast heartbeat, and weight loss, among other symptoms.

Since each person may react differently to different approaches, creating a customized treatment strategy is essential to treating this illness. A customized approach considers the distinct qualities, inclinations, and situations of every patient.

The Value Of Tailored Strategies:

1. Various Reasons for Hyperthyroidism:

• A number of underlying conditions, such as thyroiditis, toxic nodular goiter, and Graves' disease, may induce hyperthyroidism. A customized strategy is needed for each of these ailments in order to treat the unique causes of hormone overproduction.

2. Differential Symptomatology

• Each person may experience hyperthyroidism symptoms quite differently. Some people may have anxiety and weight loss, while others can have palpitations or heat intolerance. By tailoring care, medical practitioners may focus on each patient's most problematic symptoms.

3. Health History and Concomitant Conditions:

• It's critical to take into account a person's medical history and any current medical issues. For example, a patient with cardiovascular problems could need a different course of therapy than a patient without such problems.

4. Patient Lifestyle and Preferences:

• Treatment plan adherence is greatly influenced by the patient's preferences, way of life, and daily routines. By matching suggestions to a patient's values, personalized treatments increase the likelihood that the patient would follow the recommended course of action.

Collaborating With Medical Experts:

1. Comprehensive Diagnosis:

• A precise diagnosis is essential to individualized care. Thyroid function tests, imaging investigations, and blood tests are just a few of the comprehensive evaluations that medical specialists utilize to determine the precise kind and cause of hyperthyroidism.

2. Working Together to Make Decisions:

• It's critical that patients and healthcare providers collaborate when making decisions. This guarantees that the aims and values of the patient are reflected in the treatment plan, encouraging a feeling of responsibility and dedication to the management process.

3. Frequent Observation:

• Regular monitoring is required for personalized treatment programs in order to evaluate the efficacy of therapies and modify the strategy as necessary. Working closely with medical professionals enables prompt modifications depending on how the patient responds to therapy.

Creating A Network Of Support:

1. Teaching the Patient:

• A patient who is well-informed may take a more active role in their care. Giving people access to informational materials and explanations concerning hyperthyroidism, its adverse effects, and available treatments enables them to make wise choices.

2. Including Friends and Family:

• Creating a support system involves more than just medical experts; it also involves friends and family. Involving family members promotes understanding and encouragement throughout the course of therapy, helping to provide a supportive atmosphere.

3. Getting Mental Health Support Available:

• Anxiety and mood swings are two psychological effects of hyperthyroidism. It is imperative that the individualized treatment plan include mental health care.

This might include using support groups, therapy, or other mental health services.

4. Examining Lifestyle Elements:

• Lifestyle adjustments, such as dietary adjustments, exercise, and stress reduction, may support medical treatments. Creating a support system with tools for these lifestyle changes increases the treatment plan's overall efficacy.

To sum up, a customized approach to treating hyperthyroidism acknowledges the individuality of every patient and designs treatments to meet their particular requirements, preferences, and situations.

CHAPTER EIGHT

Case Studies And Success Stories

Interventions Related To Nutrition:

Case Study: A patient with hyperthyroidism investigated diet, emphasizing foods high in iodine and supplements containing selenium. With consistent follow-up, thyroid function was gradually improved, resulting in a decrease in symptoms and finally normal thyroid hormone levels for the patient.

Body-Mind Techniques:

Success Story: The patient made regular use of stress-relieving exercises like yoga and meditation. These habits seemed to help stabilize thyroid function and were eventually found to have a good effect on their general well-being.

Herbal Treatments:

Case Study: Given the possibility of their antithyroid properties, the patient chose to take herbal medicines including lemon balm and bugleweed. The patient's symptoms improved and thyroid hormone levels gradually decreased throughout routine monitoring.

Actual Experiences Using Different Methods:

Traditional Chinese Medicine (TCM) with Acupuncture:

Patient Experience: Acupuncture and Traditional Chinese Medicine (TCM) have been effective in treating hyperthyroidism symptoms for some people. The energy flow in the body is said to be rebalanced by acupuncture, and TCM herbal treatments may have adaptogenic properties.

The Functional Medicine Method:

Real-World Experience: A patient adopted a functional medicine strategy that focuses on finding and treating the underlying causes of health problems. This person reported improvements in thyroid function and a decrease in symptoms after undergoing extensive testing, dietary modifications, and lifestyle changes.

Good Results And Difficulties Faced:

Favorable Results:

Numerous people have claimed that using alternative methods has improved their symptoms of hyperthyroidism, highlighting the need for individualized treatment and comprehensive lifestyle adjustments.

A higher quality of life has been attained by some patients whose thyroid hormone levels were effectively brought within the normal range.

Problems:

Finding a strategy that works for everyone might be difficult in the absence of standardized alternative therapies for hyperthyroidism.

Different people react differently to alternative treatments, and finding the best mix of interventions may take some time.

Knowledge Gained From Patient Experiences:

Tailored Attention:

Since every person reacts to alternative methods in a different way, individualized treatment plans that cater to the patient's unique requirements and circumstances are essential.

Working together with medical professionals:

Collaboration between patients and healthcare providers is frequently necessary for successful results. It is essential to frequently monitor thyroid function and modify strategies as necessary.

Changes to a Holistic Lifestyle:

Adopting holistic lifestyle changes, such as stress reduction, dietary modifications, and mindful activities, frequently results in patients finding success.

It is important to stress that alternative medicine should be seen as an adjunct to traditional medical care, not as a substitute for it.

CHAPTER NINE

Research And Future Trends

Research And Trends In Hyperthyroidism In The Future:

1. Research on Genetics and Molecular Biology:

Gaining knowledge about the genetic foundation of hyperthyroidism may result in more individualized treatment plans.

• Studying molecular pathways may help find new medication targets for better treatment.

2. Immunotherapy:

Examining how the immune system contributes to hyperthyroidism might lead to the development of immunotherapeutic treatments.

• Immune response modulation may provide focused therapeutic approaches.

3. Environmental Factors and Epigenetics:

• Investigating how epigenetic changes and environmental influences affect thyroid function may provide insights into prophylactic actions.

4. Studies on quality of life and patient-reported outcomes:

• Assessing the effects of hyperthyroidism and its therapies on patients' quality of life may be the main focus of future studies.

• More patient-centered treatment may be directed by including patient-reported outcomes.

New Technologies And Therapies:

1. Alternatives to Radioactive Iodine:

• Research is being done to find less harmful substitutes for radioactive iodine treatment that are just as effective.

2. Specialized Treatments:

• Researching and creating medications that target hyperactive thyroid receptors, in particular, may lead to more effective and precise therapy choices.

3. Dietary strategies and nutraceuticals:

Complementary therapy techniques may result from investigating the impact of certain nutrients and dietary components in the management of hyperthyroidism.

4. Biological Interventions:

• The potential of biologics, such as monoclonal antibodies, to modify thyroid function without the negative effects of traditional therapies may be investigated.

Technology's Place In The Management Of Hyperthyroidism:

1. Remote monitoring and telemedicine:

• Telemedicine may help with patient monitoring from a distance, guaranteeing prompt medication modifications and lowering the frequency of clinic visits.

2. Diagnosis using Artificial Intelligence (AI):

• By evaluating imaging and laboratory data, AI algorithms may help with the timely and precise diagnosis of hyperthyroidism.

3. Wearable Technology:

• Wearable technology can monitor symptoms and vital signs, giving patients and medical professionals access to real-time data.

4. Digital Health Resources:

• Patient education, medication adherence, and patient-provider communication may all be facilitated by integrated digital platforms.

Present Studies And Encouragering Advancements:

1. Agonists and Antagonists of the Thyroid Hormone Receptor:

• Research is still being done to create new thyroid hormone receptor agonists and antagonists for more specialized and efficient care.

2. Immunostimulatory Medication:

• The goal of immunomodulatory medication research is to control the immunological response in hyperthyroidism, perhaps providing an alternative to current therapeutic approaches.

3. Treatments Based on MicroRNA:

• Researching the activity of microRNAs in the thyroid may help create treatments that adjust the expression of certain genes in hyperthyroidism.

4. Eco-friendly Nanoparticles:

• Targeted delivery of thyroid-inhibiting drugs with minimal side effects on other tissues is being investigated using nanotechnology.

In conclusion, interdisciplinary approaches combining genetics, immunology, and cutting-edge technology for more accurate diagnosis and therapy are anticipated to be the future trends in hyperthyroidism research. Along with further research, emerging medicines and technology have the potential to improve patient outcomes and improve the overall management of hyperthyroidism. Always seek the counsel of medical specialists for the most up-to-date information and customized recommendations.

Conclusion

In summary, the multimodal approach of the simple solution approach to hyperthyroidism includes medication, lifestyle changes, and patient education. A thorough approach to managing hyperthyroidism is crucial since it is recognized as a complicated disorder with several contributing causes such as hereditary predispositions, immunological difficulties, and hormone imbalances.

Summary Of The Main Ideas:

1. Medical Intervention: Antithyroid drugs, radioactive iodine treatment, and, in some situations, surgery are among the medical interventions often used to treat hyperthyroidism. The goals of these treatments are to control thyroid hormone levels and reduce symptoms. Customizing treatment programs to each patient's requirements requires close monitoring and cooperation with medical specialists.

2. Lifestyle Adjustments: Adjusting one's lifestyle is a major part of controlling hyperthyroidism. Having a nutritionally dense, low-iodine diet that is well-balanced may promote thyroid health. In addition to improving general well-being, stress

reduction practices, consistent exercise, and enough sleep may also have a favorable effect on thyroid function. It's also a good idea to stay away from triggers like excessive coffee and tobacco usage.

3.   Empowering patients with hyperthyroidism entails giving them the information and resources they need to take an active role in their own treatment. Patients are more equipped to make choices when they are educated about their disease, available treatments, and possible lifestyle changes. Online forums and support groups may provide a forum for people to exchange stories and learn from others facing comparable difficulties.

4. Frequent Monitoring: Blood tests and physical examinations are essential for frequent monitoring due to the dynamic nature of thyroid function. This makes it possible to rapidly address any changes in thyroid hormone levels and modify treatment strategies as necessary. Effective long-term management requires cooperative communication between patients and healthcare professionals.

Providing Hyperthyroid People With Empowerment:

Helping people with hyperthyroidism requires a multifaceted strategy that goes beyond prescription drugs. It consists of:

1. Education: Giving people thorough information on hyperthyroidism's origins, symptoms, and available treatments

encourages them to take an active role in choosing their medical care. Gaining knowledge about the significance of medication compliance and lifestyle adjustments promotes a feeling of control over the illness.

2. Self-Monitoring: Encouraging people to keep an eye on their symptoms and routinely check their vital indicators, such as their heart rate, may help identify any changes in thyroid function early on. Proactive contact with healthcare practitioners and prompt modifications to treatment programs are made possible by this self-awareness.

3. Support Networks: People with hyperthyroidism may connect with others going through similar struggles by creating

or joining support networks and online forums. In addition to offering emotional support, sharing experiences, coping mechanisms, and success stories may provide useful insights into the day-to-day management of the illness.

Considering The Future Of Treatment For Hyperthyroidism:

Thanks to technological and scientific improvements in medicine, the treatment of hyperthyroidism has a bright future. Important things to think about in the future are:

1. Personalized Medicine: Further investigation into the biochemical and genetic causes of hyperthyroidism may

result in more individualized therapeutic strategies. Customizing therapies according to each patient's genetic profile and biomarkers may increase the effectiveness of therapy and reduce adverse effects.

2. Digital Health Solutions: Real-time thyroid function and general health monitoring may be made easier with the incorporation of digital health technology, such as wearables and smartphone apps. With the use of these tools, patients may take charge of their health and provide medical professionals with useful information for individualized treatment regimens.

3. Therapies Innovations: Continued research may lead to the discovery of new

therapy modalities, such as innovative drugs with reduced adverse effects and increased effectiveness. Examining complementary and alternative therapy may increase the alternatives open to people with hyperthyroidism.

4. Improved Patient Education: New developments in communication and instructional platforms have the potential to improve patient education even further. For those with hyperthyroidism, interactive and user-friendly materials like virtual reality and augmented reality apps may provide immersive educational opportunities.

In conclusion, more individualized, patient-centered therapy backed by cutting-edge technology is what the future of hyperthyroidism treatment promises. Increasing people's awareness, giving them a feeling of control, and using cutting-edge medical innovations would help people with hyperthyroidism manage their condition better and live better.

THE END